NEXT LEVEL TEACHING- BEYOND PANDEMIC 2020

"MOVING FORWARD - EYES WIDE OPEN"

Viola L. Grays-Wiley

WESTBOW PRESS®
A DIVISION OF THOMAS NELSON & ZONDERVAN

WestBow Press books may be ordered through booksellers or by contacting:

WestBow Press
A Division of Thomas Nelson & Zondervan
1663 Liberty Drive
Bloomington, IN 47403
www.westbowpress.com
1 (866) 928-1240

ISBN: 978-1-9736-9827-2 (sc)
ISBN: 978-1-9736-9829-6 (hc)
ISBN: 978-1-9736-9828-9 (e)

Library of Congress Control Number: 2020913564

Print information available on the last page.

WestBow Press rev. date: 08/05/2020

DEDICATION

MRS. FANNIE MAE GRAYS

Always honoring the winds beneath

my wings, for teaching

me about caring, the importance

of family, life-long

learning, and bridges built through education.

CONTENTS

ACKNOWLEDGEMENTS

First and foremost, I want to take this opportunity to acknowledge the Creator of the Universe. He gives me the passion to keep fighting for equity in education for all children. Many children don't realize that they have a right to quality education, regardless of the color of their skin, racial or ethnic background, physical or mental disability, ELL and ESL deficits, deprived demographic location, apartment building, or suburban residential status. This lights the fire within my soul to push forward for every child and every student, enhancing the entire professional learning community. It's all about the students.

I'm deeply concerned for any child who wakes up in the morning without a dream at heart, in the United States of America, or in any nation across the globe, because dreams build character. Character builds purpose. From the east coast to the west coast, from the north side to the south side of your cities, in the rural areas of this country that are so often overlooked and mismanaged, from sea to shining sea, I write this book for children, parents, teachers, school administrators, school boards, politicians, religious leaders, elected officials, and all who can and will make a positive difference in the lives of children.

To my Family- My Dad, Tarri, Jay, Meech, Annie, Debteen, Darlene, Mary, Vickey, Terry, DD,

Tommie, Chris, Roger, Milton, Tarrianna, Genesis, Emma-Grace, Elijah, Jakwon, Malachi, Valenique, Tiffany, TJ, Treasuir, KK, Miah, JJ, Marilyn, Dr.Timothy Holston, JR, D-Man, Josiah, JW, Aunt Ida Mae Thomas & Family, Aunt Emma Lee Smith & Family, and Uncle Joshua Smith & Family, Evangelist Sandra Taylor, Ella Chandler, Ruthie Peoples-Hampton, Shirley Crigler-Livingston, Mary Smith-Brown, JoanneThomas-Wiley, Dr.Tameka Ivory-Walls, Aaron Wilson & the Wilson Singers, the Granderson & Smith Families, Dr. Jennifer Young-Wallace & the Delaney Family, Mrs. Faye Naylor, Doris. Powell, Ada Meeks, Jennifer H-Mathis, and Mayor Ajoku of Cruger, MS

Dr. Frankie Swoope-Bynum and Orlando Ceaser serve as inspiration and continue to provide positive and powerful influences on my professional growth;

Respected professional colleagues -Dr. Cynthia Levy, Mrs. Carole Davis, Dr. M. Karen Jones, students and Staff at JWLA & BOLA, IL SD 152.5, CCH SD 160, Fran Arvia, Marie Nisbeth, LaTonya Walker, Muriel M-Holliman, Pamela Jaeger, Sandy Sebastian, Vivian Washington, Monique W-Shepard, Angelica Faith, Michelle Harris, Danielle Thomaston, Laurie & Barbara Oliver, Dorissa Woodland, Sabrina Williams, Mr. & Mrs. Albert Harrison and Amanda Elzy Elementary & High Schools- Greenwood, MS; Vaiden High School, in Carroll County (MS) and Holmes County Schools (MS)

My Pandemic 2020 New Teachers/ Mentees-(IL School District 152.5): Mrs Halper, Mrs. Paprocki, Ms. Foster, Mrs. Zeimetz, Ms Lusby, Ms Kelman, Ms. Mistina, Ms. O'Dell, Mrs. George, Mrs. Dowdy, Ms. Oliver, Ms. McNicholas, Mrs. Martin,

Ms Strange, Ms Booth, Mrs. Pickett, Mrs. Johnson, Mrs. Szychlinski, Ms. Cochran, Mrs. Henderson … SUPER TEACHERS!!!

Abounding Life COGIC - Bishop Ocie Booker & Family, Mother Earnestine Adams, Dr. Jane Crosley & the Adams Family, Elder Verner & Family, Elder Harris & Family, the late Mother Howze, Mother Knight, Mother Mack, Greg Owens & Family, Zoriante Brown & Family, Gwen Gray, Dr. C. Williams, and Annette Knownas ANET

Finally, I would be remiss if I didn't recognize all the teachers across the United States of America who stepped up without missing a beat, to providing remote learning to America's students having access to technology, as well as the underprivileged students who had to have a less advanced method of contact and communication. These phenomenal teachers did whatever they had to do to make sure the achievement gap was not widened under their watch. On behalf of all the educators, I respectfully say, "THANK YOU, TEACHERS!"

ABOUT THE AUTHOR

Viola Grays -Wiley attended Amanda Elzy High School, where she developed a rich background in music, under the leadership of the renowned Mr. Albert C. Harrison. It was at this school that she crafted her skill of organizing and assembling pitch-perfect vocal choirs and groups all across the states of Mississippi, Tennessee, and later in the state of Illinois. As a member of the Amanda Elzy Concert Choir, she sang alto and performed at colleges and universities across the South, capturing audiences with their smooth, distinctive a'capella selections. Several gospel groups she coordinated, and/or is affiliated with, are still performing today. One in particular, the Grays Singer of Black Hawk, Mississippi, is her family's group. Distinctively, a key fact to be noted back then, her oratorical skills began to surface. It was clear there was more to come!

She received her baccalaureate in Elementary Education from Mississippi Valley State University, in Itta Bena, Mississippi (an HBCU). She further studied literacy education at Mississippi State University, located in Mississippi State, Mississippi. Later, she completed additional studies of reading and literacy at Portland State University and then at the University of Chicago. However, it was during her work at Portland State University where she underwent a teaching paradigm shift. This afforded her the opportunity to work in partnership with Dr. Kent Johnson and Morningside Learning Systems within a number of Chicago Public Schools. It was during this enlightenment that she was introduced to the late and great Dr. Ogden Lindsley. She became a protege of Dr. Lindsley, the "Father of Precision Teaching", who introduced her as keynote speaker at the 1997 Annual Behavior Analysis International Convention at the Hyatt Regency in Chicago. Dr. Lindsley so eloquently introduced her as "The Teacher's teacher". In her roles as a classroom teacher, lead literacy teacher, department chairperson, state professional development provider, state quality review team member, school principal, active member of the American Federation of Teachers, National Education Association, Illinois Education Association, voted "WHO'S WHO AMONG AMONG AMERICA'S TEACHERS" five consecutive years, nothing has been more rewarding than years of outstanding student achievement, not just on state mandated assessments, but daily in classrooms where she has taught. As a graduate student at Chicago State University, she rededicated herself to history by studying at "The Teachers' College", as it was once known. Here she received a solid foundation for reaching within herself to advocate for removing disparities in education for all children. What a dynamic motivational speaker she is! The author has always felt that when students excel, she has succeeded. She further quotes, "If I want to know if my students are learning, I can always ask them. Dr. Lindsley taught me this. Thanks, Og!" This simple strategy has stood the test of time in her more than thirty-five years in classrooms across the country!

INTRODUCTION

What does the phrase "Return to Normalcy" mean to you? Well, to me it signifies getting back to living the way I was prior to the Pandemic of 2020. But really? Can we ever truly go back to life at that level? Will school-aged children ever realistically go back to pre-pandemic status mentally, socially, or emotionally? I would always hope that present conditions in schools will have a blanket of support for students, teachers, and staff, that is most definitely therapeutic. *Disclaimer: The author in no way attempts to provide medical advice, nor has medical background. All medical concerns should be directed to your health care provider.*

What I am trying to say is this entire ordeal or presence of COVID-19, has affected individuals in life at every possible plateau. Unless we begin again with a full court of wrap-around services, we will not move forward stronger together. Once school designs have been enhanced to include staff supports- mentally, socially, and emotionally, then those staff members will be able to provide sustainable instructional practices that will positively impact teaching and learning. "... Education has a moral purpose ... to make a difference in the lives of students, regardless of background" (Fullan, 1991).

This book, NEXT LEVEL TEACHING-BEYOND PANDEMIC 2020, is intended to steer mindsets towards recalibrating the players on the field. We can't make a refreshing change until we begin to converse about what we care about. More dialogue must begin in our schools and professional learning communities. But these conversations can't be opaque. They must be transparent and far-reaching.

Discussions must not continue to fall on silent ears. For example, how should we measure success in the classroom? What does teacher - student relationships look like in the classroom? Where is the classroom? What new role can parents expect to be involved in inside the parameters of educating their children? In other words, using reflections based on what we know, how can a closer connection emerge just in case traditional schooling is abruptly halted, but due to proactive communication, students lose very little downtime because parents and guardians are kept abreast of learning goals and standards for their children BECAUSE OF the pandemic?

In other words, guidelines should be written in both traditional and remote learning formats. This would be so beneficial because if we vertically align our goals and standards so that no matter where students are enrolled in school in the United States of America, they will not fall behind. After the pandemic, this is the global edge that we need. In fact, every country has to reshape its educational design to fit this format. America will simply be the leader!

Here is an example of what I'm referring to. Let's look at third grade. Given the normal 180-days school calendar, on the 47th day of the school year, all 3rd graders will work on LANGUAGE ARTS- Subject/Verb Agreement, MATHEMATICS- Adding Fractions, SOCIAL STUDIES- Pilgrims and Native Americans, SCIENCE/STEM EDUCATION -Static Electricity annd Balloons. Our goal has to become "LEARNING FOR ALL: WHATEVER IT TAKES" (Lezotte, 1997, p.2)

So, no matter what the physical location for the child is, the skills and goals will not change. Children appreciate routines, even more than adults. It is astoundingly rewarding to a child to know what they will be learning and why. On the remote learning and traditional curricula, teachers could explicitly input skills students need to master and why they need to master the skills at a particular time. Transparency! Therefore, as students enroll in whatever school at their respective grade levels, they will remain on tract for college and career readiness.

In cases of extreme weather conditions, pandemics, any Act of God, when schools must be closed, students and parents can rest assured because they could visit their schools 'websites and default to eLearning Plans for their respective schools and grade levels, then continue progressing academically. This, my friends, is NEXT LEVEL TEACHING-BEYOND PANDEMIC 2020.

CHAPTER 1

STARTING OVER

I can only speak to the catastrophic pandemic of 2020 for myself, as a teacher, parent, daughter, educational consultant, community resident, and a member of society at large. I begin by asking myself a plethora of questions. How are teachers supposed to return to a state of normalcy after a pandemic? What does that look like? What will it mean for students, parents, grandparents, and guardians? Where does safety and security begin or end? How will support staff begin to address the new multitude of social and emotional issues that probably have evolved, while continuing to address earlier problems that existed prior to the pandemic? What does the welcome-back-to-school staff meeting look like for school administrators? What will the next memorandum from the State Board of Education include? Should remote learning be embedded in regular school curricula as a standby tool, just in case more craziness sporadically reappears?

Individuals around the globe are panicking with inquiry. But most importantly, this time decision makers want to use knowledge from this event to make wise decisions moving forward. Those in charge want to operate at an unprecedented level of preparedness. However, there is no handbook available that will provide adequate fundamental strategies for recreating an entire country's educational system after a pandemic at the magnitude recently experienced here in the United States and around the world.

One can only hope and pray that communities of individuals, having sound minds and resiliency, will rebuild based on what they know, and aspire to create schools and classrooms that embark upon the fundamental theme of being better and stronger together.

The best way to start over is to glance back. If we gleaned nothing else from the arrival of COVID-19, one thing we should have mastered quite well is the art of reflecting. In my mind, I thought daily about where I was in my life. What should I have done differently prior to the onset of the pandemic? What could I have done better? How will I be better when this event is in the history books and life is returning to some level of normalcy?

Oh yes—we have had time to reflect since the *stay-at-home orders* were given. I believe, deep down inside, most of us spent an enormous amount of time reflecting, probably without even realizing that this was what was occurring. A reflection is a positive energy waiting to be dispersed. It's a good thing. Only when you are able to make sense of your past, can you accelerate into your future. However, before we move forward, we must recognize and acknowledge mentally and physically that we must *start over.* What this means is—life as we knew it simply does not exist anymore.

After work, I had time to spend on Facebook connecting with audiences. Many times, the coronavirus was the trending conversation, of course.

Parents began to reach out to teachers thanking them for their support during the school year. There were even times when parents were screaming, "I need help!" or "Stay home because my kids need to go back to school!" Whether in the spirit of humor or reality, many parents developed a new appreciation for teachers. These social media conversations are continuing throughout the duration of the pandemic. This was the initial phase of a new beginning for parent–teacher dialogue, real connections that were reciprocal.

You see, this monster virus was larger than any creature students had viewed at the movies or on cable TV, yet the enemy was invisible. The true dynamics are quite surreal. We all know that some movies are rated too severe or extreme for young audiences, yet our youngest audience members were not exempt from COVID 19.

Communication begins the healing process. You've got to talk about where we are. Then we can map out where we want to be. Next step, let's talk about how we can get there. Remember, when we set goals and develop a mission and vision, we can get there more expeditiously and efficiently while working together. This should be a lesson well-learned from the pandemic of 2020. As a classroom teacher, I've learned through experience that if I can reach students, then I can teach them. Conversations start the process.

Looking back at where America's schools were prior to this historic event will cause us as a nation to zoom in on *the-hows* and *the-whys* of everyday operations and become more insightful individuals. Yes, we're all learning a lot. The insights we have acquired from actually surviving an epidemic of this magnitude when we were undaunted has given us an inner strength to move forward with perseverance. Yes. we will survive!

To start over, we must look within ourselves to pull from this energy a spirit of relentless determination. Know that we can make it. Yes, we will be stronger together. We learned to lean on one another from one community to the next. This spirit of resolve will allow America to thrive again. We must remain cognizant of our goals and timely reallocate resources sufficiently.

We can't just start over for the sake of starting over. We must be strategic about every step we take, considering what we know. It behooves us to function with the mindset that we are all connected for the greater good of our communities. New operation manuals must be devised to include all entities, so there will not be disparities from one racial group to the other. Expectations of success for all students must become the norm.

Creative ways of reaching out to students should be welcomed by school administrators. This paradigm shift will not happen overnight because the pandemic is lasting dreadfully longer than an overnight ordeal. Nevertheless, many of the disparities students face in education started long, long ago, even before *Brown v Board of Education*. Let me clarify for my young readers and students of color who may be wondering what is *Brown v Board of Education*? In the United States, a number of African American plaintiffs led by Oliver Brown filed a class-action lawsuit against the Board of Education of Topeka, Kansas, in 1951, because Mr. Brown's daughter was denied entrance to Topeka's all-white schools. This case proceeded to the United

States Supreme Court in 1952. The Supreme Court combined four other related school segregation cases into a single case, which came to be known as *Brown v Board of Education of Topeka*.

Thurgood Marshall served as chief attorney for the plaintiffs. After two years before the courts for hearings, the Supreme Court ruled unanimously that racial segregation of children in public schools was unconstitutional. So, today black, white, and brown students can attend ANY public school in the country. One step forward! This is the magnitude of changes that must occur after COVID-19, This case served as a platform for the civil rights activists in their quest to rid the United States of inequities in education. Unfortunately, so much work still urgently needs to be done in this area today. Thirteen years after this historic Supreme Court ruling, President

Lyndon B. Johnson appointed Thurgood Marshall as the first African American Supreme Court justice in America.

This should serve as a catalyst for America's school systems to move forward strategically. How can we improve unless we know where we've been? The pandemic of 2020 appeared at our doorsteps unannounced and certainly unwelcomed. We must rise from this disaster. We can't let it define who we are. We must use hindsight to give us foresight. One thing we can be certain of moving forward is the affirmation that we will be better and stronger together.

We will use technology in unprecedented ways, but it is only one vital tool within an arsenal of many. Human connections and productive relationships will formulate atmospheres of inquiry. Students will be taught to think critically daily. Problem-solving will present the foundation for most of our school lessons and activities. There will be students who learn differently and at varying rates. So let's think about the new shift of education.

Here's a sample of a question we may find ourselves pondering. Should students move with the group and remain at level 3 skills when they are absolutely ready for level 4? These are the kinds of fruitful questions that must be addressed by policymakers to move our country toward the top. Sometimes we have the individuals restrained due to formalities. They may have the ideology, the strategy, the cure, the next engineering innovation, but are held back due to archaic educational laws or guidelines. A new frontier has evolved! We must train our brains to think new thoughts incessantly and cooperatively.

Next level teaching is outside the box *---Totally Outside*!:

Grow from What You Know!

CHAPTER 2

LOOKING BACK TO MOVE AHEAD

This caused me to go way back, all the way back to the *one-room schoolhouses*. Let's take a look. I'm inquisitive. Traditional schools are so different today from the way they were in the days of the one-room schoolhouses. Earlier in our country's history, all of the students gathered in a single room for learning. One teacher taught every grade level of elementary students. What did that look like?

Well, for one thing, you were in a classroom with

your sisters, brothers, cousins, their sisters, brothers, your neighbor's school-aged elementary children with their siblings, and so forth. The students ranged from first through eighth grade! Just the thought of this today, and all I can say is, "Wow!" Everybody in one room with one overseer! Again, the thought is mind-boggling!

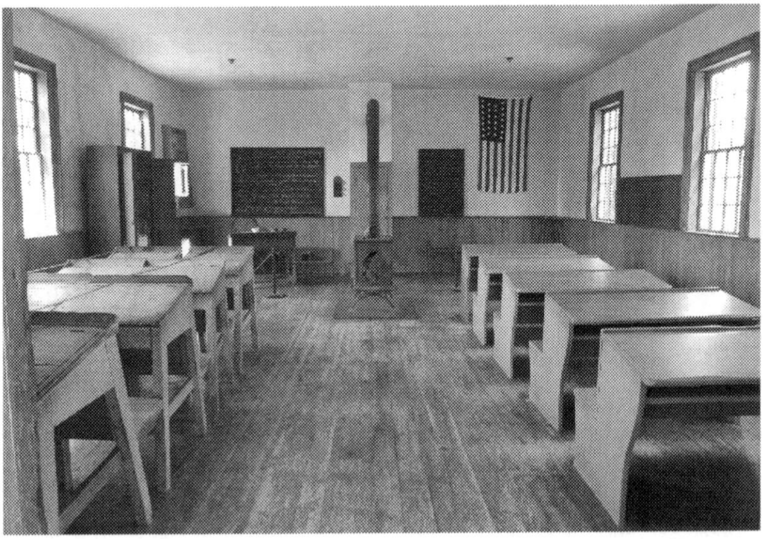

What did this *one teacher* teach? Well, the teacher usually taught reading, writing, arithmetic, history, and geography. However, more focus was on the first three—reading, 'riting, and 'rithmetic —which came to be known as the 3 R's. In the winter, there was no central heating unit. The teacher and students had to build a fire in a fireplace or cast-iron stove or heater.

Still all the students showed up on time or early for learning. In the summer, there was no central air conditioning. Yes, it was hot! They opened windows and used fans made from paper or boxes. And, yes, they still were eager to learn all they could before the long journey home on foot sometimes in the rain, burning sunshine, sleet, snow, or stormy weather.

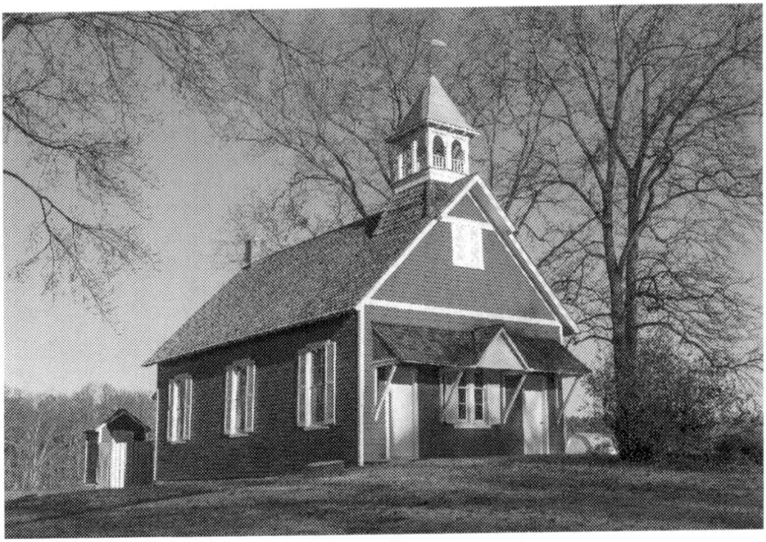

CHAPTER 3

LEARNING BY ANY MEANS NECESSARY

The teacher and the students just had to make it work, whatever the condition of the weather. The students just wanted to learn all they could as the teacher taught everyone at the same time in one room. They wanted an education by any means necessary---no inside bathrooms, no electricity, no school buses, no cars or trucks.

Yes, most children walked to school or rode horses and wagons. Still, they learned anyway. When we hear the poem or song "Mary had a little lamb who followed her to school one day" … perhaps there is some truth to the words of the song.

Teachers and students did all of their own cleaning. Students learned to be responsible just by doing … through osmosis. They learned respect just by seeing it in action at school, day in and day out. The younger children learned a lot from the older students in class. After all, they were all in the same room.

It's just amazing to me that back then, there were so few discipline problems in the one-room schoolhouse. How did ONE TEACHER maintain order and disperse knowledge simultaneously, while academic achievement continued to rise?

How did these one-room schoolhouse teachers reach and teach so many students at varying cognitive and developmental levels without a school board, local school counsel, superintendent, assistant superintendent, principal, assistant principal, school social worker, school psychologist, speech therapist, lunchroom supervisor, director of special education services, school security guard, school secretary, truant officer, dean of students, etc.? This is truly bewildering to me.

Today, in the year 2020, where are we going wrong? Prior to the Pandemic, discipline problems were so rampant that many highly qualified teachers were unable to teach. Through no fault of their own, dedicated teachers were caught up in a system where they almost had no where to turn to. The disruptive students were made to look innocent by school board policies. Where are we off point? There must be a sign somewhere that we are missing---a GPS that hasn't been programmed correctly, an email that went to the wrong inbox, what is it?

Well, when I visualize what occurred in the one-room schoolhouses, I must acknowledge that the physical journey to and from the school building must carry significant weight. You see if you grew up living in rural Mississippi, as I did, you understood how to ride the bus to school and back home peacefully, without distracting the bus driver. I was thrilled to ride and not have to walk 20-25 miles to school, whereas, I had siblings who had to struggle to get to school because the cut-off location of the bus route didn't extend to where we lived. You just learned to appreciate opportunities in life.

For that reason alone, I knew how to ride the bus and not cause problems for the bus driver. However, our new journey to school may simply be out of the bedroom and into the living room on the sofa or sitting at the dining room table. We must make a large shift in our thinking … BEYOND PANDEMIC 2020!!!

CHAPTER 4

CONDITIONED FOR LEARNING

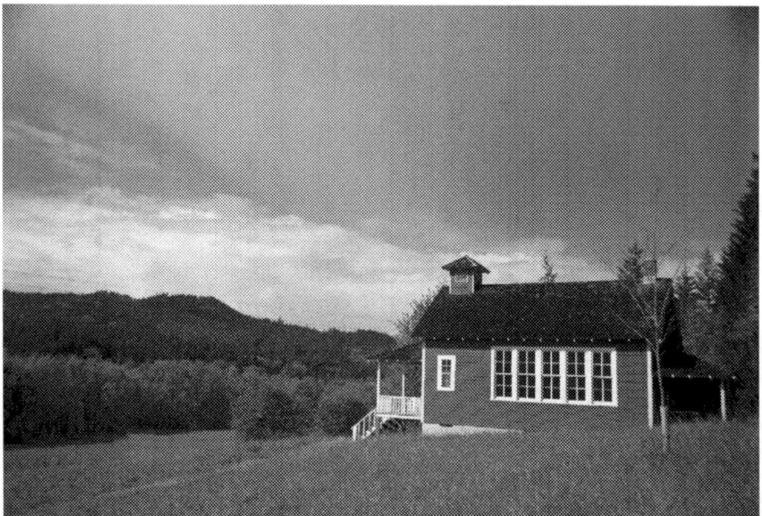

Many of the one-room schoolhouses also served as churches or places where the community could gather, if necessary. Truly remarkable! Just look at the maximum utilization of resources for the common good of all. Nothing was wasted. Clothes, shoes, toys---were all recycled through the families and communities. Whenever there was an abundance of eggs, they were shared with the neighbors … peas, beans, corn, watermelons, tomatoes... You name it!!! Community was about Unity!

People were conditioned to work together. I am not saying that America was a nation without its problems. There was discrimination, segregation, inequalities, and injustices that would consume this entire book and many more that haven't been, but need to be written, about history before and since the Civil War in the United States of America.

However, my focus is the structure of delivery and mastery of instruction, without the obstacle of classroom disruptions. How were student so engaged in the learning process without the availability of support staff? How can we as a nation get to a level once again where we produce student populations who are thirsty for knowledge? This new blended learning may provide the quest for knowledge that existed in the one-room school houses.

Blended learning should open doors and close disparities in education. Everyone has to become accountable to progress. Students, parents, teachers, school administrators, school boards, elected officials, and support staff, everyone working together will get us to where we are trying to go. At the end of the day, it will all boil down to state and federal funding, in the hands of lawmakers. For sure, they must step up and do their part. The pandemic only made prevalent inequities in education more apparent.

Technology within itself is an added level of support that is available in a number of schools across the country, but not nearly enough. The pandemic only made this information more transparent. Furthermore, according to the National Education Association, about 8.5 -12 million school-aged students don't have access to the internet. These disparities in educating students are unimaginable!

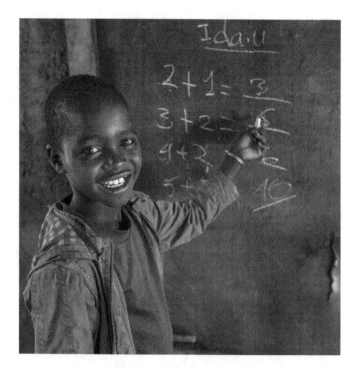

Prior to the pandemic, in many classrooms, some teachers were saying you can't say a word to youngsters about anything. They say some students talk back to adults without hesitation. Oh, somebody, please bring me a one-room schoolhouse! Is it that some students have access to more of what they DON'T need and maybe they are not aware of what they DO need? I'm beginning to feel like less would be more profitable for some of our youths in society today. This is not to promote disparities in education in any way. I just feel that we can't allow ourselves, as parents and teachers, to become disconnected from our youths. One philosophy I am definitely sure of is that if we can't reach them, we can't teach them, whether traditional or remote learning. So that leads me to the concepts of connections and sensitivity.

It is more critical than ever to build relationships.

This was commonplace in the one-room schoolhouse. Everyone connected on a daily basis. Now technology has instituted itself between personal interactions with families and friends. It is normal to not look up to acknowledge an adult walking into the room with many electronic gadgets in the hands of youths, and not interact with any human being for 24-48, maybe even 72 hours. This wedge of isolation is growing every day. Because of this disconnect, people, especially the very young, are hurting more and more. No technology will ever replace the need for human-to-human connections.

CHAPTER 5

BUILDING RELATIONSHIPS

Technology does not replace the physical need to build constructive relationships with others. Adults and children want to belong. There is a social-emotional need to belong in society. Young people are craving for meaningful relationships. I feel that the one-room schoolhouse provided an over - arching feeling of belonging. Just as the mother hen nurtures her young, these gifted one-room schoolhouse teachers had immeasurable talents to give students the feeling of safety and structure for social and cognitive development, simultaneously, in a family environment.

Now that I am witnessing and enduring the Coronavirus Global Pandemic, and schools have been shutdown, I keep seeing reminders of the One-room Schoolhouse. Teachers are engaging in what is known as "eLearning", to connect with and engage students. This simply means electronically connecting with students instead of in-person direct contact. I feel that more parents have a greater visualization of the teacher's daily plight, since the students are being home-schooled along with teacher- directed and supported eLearning or remote learning activities.

There are quite a few parents reaching out to social media saying "This is too much! I can't do this!" Most of the time they are referring to is time spent reviewing eLearning materials with the child, or spending family time when the regular school day would have been over. It is understandably a monumental task. Just dealing with the requirements of surviving the pandemic is an enormous responsibility without having to take care of the educational home structure for children. This would be overwhelming for the average person.

One doctrine that seems to prevail in traditional schools, as well as in remote learning, is high expectations yielding positive results. You probably have heard the old joke about the substitute teacher of a group of high school students labeled as underachievers or at-risk. It puzzled the school's principal when those students scored very well on the state assessment.

Through questioning the substitute about what strategies she used to get such phenomenal scores from this group of students, the substitute said that she knew they would score high when she saw their IQ scores next to their names on the roster. "What IQ scores?" The principal replied, "Those weren't their IQ scores ... those were their locker numbers!"

There are quite a few messages embedded within that joke, but I think you'll agree that the overarching moral is to set high expectations, regardless of the task or group. You see, I can insinuate that this substitute teacher probably addressed the students as star students. She possibly taught them as a teacher of gifted students. In other words, the students felt as though the sky was the limit and they responded as stars.

With any group of humans you want to connect with, you must start by building relationships. Whatever method becomes necessary to query the audience to determine likes and dislikes, this is vital in your framework of connectivity. You can look at followings on social media. People don't follow someone unless they like them first. Maybe you'll have a few curious prowlers, but after a bit, they'll drop off, and' you'll be left with your true followers. You see, you can't wait for other people to start building relationships for you. Every day provides new opportunities for building relationships.

I remember working at a school where a newly hired lead administrator acquired a list of all staff' members' birth dates upon her arrival. This school principal would have a birthday cake and breakfast treats to honor each staff member for their respective birthdays. Did she get off to a great start? Yes, she did. Did teachers comply with her new order of business? Yes, they did happily. She came in building relationships. Her method may not be identical to yours, but gather your own creative strategies for connecting with students, staff, or audiences you want to impact. Just be sure you are not out of touch.

It's always important to reach out to students before you make any attempt to teach a lesson. Connect First! Reach them, then teach them. Here's a sample teacher or parent daily check-in:

(Especially after a traumatic event such as a pandemic!)

DAILY CHECK-IN PULSE READER

(1- 5) 1= Worst 5= Best

1. How was your night? Did you sleep okay?

2. Was breakfast okay?

3. What have you been doing for fun during free time?

4. How are you feeling right now at this very moment ?

5. Outside of school, how are you doing?

6. Is there anything you want to share?

7. Is there anything I should know?

8. "YOU ARE IMPORTANT TO ME!!! I WANT YOU TO KNOW THAT YOU TRULY MATTER TO ME!.". … (Teacher or Parent)

CHAPTER 6

MODELS FOR SCHOOLS MOVING FORWARD

Moving beyond the unforeseen crisis that America and the world is facing, our schools, teachers, students and their parents must return to a state of somewhat normalcy, so they say. Unfortunately, after a Global Pandemic, there is no road map, but I do believe, we are resilient and we will emerge stronger together. However, I do feel that this country and many others, will be new countries, where we will not take things for granted, and children who have survived this disastrous event will have a new appreciation for parents, teachers, and communities. We will move forward with our EYES WIDE OPEN. That is my dream!

Even more, parents and teachers will develop better relationships, and likewise, teachers and students will build new relationships, that will transcend into more teaching and learning in the classroom. There will be a new wave of positive interactions in the classrooms because of the turmoil that we as a country are enduring. This pandemic not only happened to teachers. It also happened to parents. But not only to parents, it happened to students. We developed a new connectivity.

There is a chain of connections and relationships that have been manifested subconsciously among us. Channeling this manifestation into positive relationships will be the quest of every educator in classrooms across the globe. Can it become a reality? I am one individual who believes not only that it can happen, but it should happen. You see true learning never reaches a plateau where we have arrived.

Authentic learning is a continuous process. Schools realize they need to have a vision in order to set goals to achieve (Wiley, 2020). Do I learn something new everyday? You bet cha! I don't desire to know it all, but my mission is to keep learning. So, as these new relationships begin to evolve, so will encountering new inquiries, brighter discoveries, better strategies, and more ways to solve problems, because of better relationships between teachers and students in classrooms.

When will schools really get a "green light" to reopen? Well, before America makes that determination, we must use a whole lot of science, and just as much common sense, considering what we do know about the virus that nearly shut the world down. We want to make sure buildings are sanitized before the arrival of staff or students. This habit of sanitizing and re-sanitizing has to become commonplace throughout the duration of the school day. It will become commonplace to re-sanitize classrooms 3-5 times per day. Any area or materials touched by staff or students, should be cleaned frequently. This includes school buses. Playgrounds should probably be closed, unless designated areas are available, whereas at least 6 feet of personal space is allowed per student (8-10 students per playground period), then playground equipment must be sanitized prior to arrival of next group. For lunch, cafeterias probably should be closed or set up with partitions for small classes of students, with majority of students remaining in classrooms, similar to lunch delivery for field trips. Until there is a vaccine or cure, **field trips** should be increased, but **all should be virtual!**

How will students and staff enter the building daily? It's makes sense to me, considering what we know, to have entry temperature checks by school nurses. There is some high tech equipment being created that checks temperatures as you enter facilities. This may become commonplace in schools. Every school will undoubtedly need at least two licensed school nurses. In addition, a staffed urgent medical care station has to be located within each building for students or staff who may present possible virus symptoms. In case of a possible virus infection, schools will need to isolate the ill immediately. Next, school will need to close for 2-3 days for thorough cleaning and sanitizing. The infected staff member or student will follow guidelines from the Center for Disease Control (CDC) before returning to the school. A close relationship must be maintained with the local health department. Remember, EYES WIDE OPEN! However, privacy guidelines must be adhered to throughout this process.

Oh, yes, we must be wondering if we should wear masks at school. The present guidance leaves us with the knowledge that face coverings for all school staff and students make perfect sense to me. Therefore, making sure that anyone entering schools wear face coverings seems to be the responsible and logical protocol to follow. However, this needs to be analyzed according to a community's infectious disease positivity rate. This should probably be advised and determined through your local health departments.

Just as we have been informed during this pandemic, special attention and concern should be given to individuals over the age of 65, as well as staff or students with underlying health conditions. Yet, privacy is extremely important.

Whenever possible, schools should limit large crowds. Perhaps, the **3 W's** will be a useful tool in regards to student and staff entry and movement within the building:

1. **Wear Mask**
2. **Wash Hands**
3. **Watch Distance**

Also, SCHOOL BELLS could alert re-sanitizing classrooms, as well as new class period.

SOCIAL DISTANCING WILL BE THE DRIVING FORCE BEHIND EVERYTHING HAPPENING INSIDE OF OR NEAR SCHOOLS! THIS will be the NEW NORMAL!

This may mean some students will start later than others. Likewise, some may return home at different times. What this really means is arrivals and dismissals may not be the same for all students. Times may need to be broken down within the framework of careful scheduling.

There will be a number of models for schools to experiment with. Because of unprecedented times, the best models are yet to be recognized. Here are a few samples I came up with on the following pages.

MODEL 1

AM Classes PM Classes

PreK-2	50%	50%
Gr 3-5	50%	50%
LUNCH PERIOD	-First Lunch	Second Lunch (arrival)
Gr 6-8	50%	50%

*Breakfast pre-bagged/ issued at Dismissal (Remote Learning→ 50%Support)

....

MODEL 2

$EMESTER ONE (SEMESTER TWO groups flip)

50% Traditional

50% Remote Learning

PreK - 2		
Gr3-5		
LUNCH PERIOD		

Gr 6-8		
Gr 9-12		

*Breakfast same as above

....

Teachers A, B, C, D, E Teachers F, G, H, I, J

MODEL 3 10- 15 students max 10-15 students max

Prek -2		
Gr 3-5		
Gr 6-8		
Gr. 9-12	REMOTE LEARNING	REMOTE LEARNING

**Nutritional Curbside Meals- Breakfast, Lunch & afternoon snacks

MODEL 4- TOTAL REMOTE LEARNING (All Grades)**

This MODEL should be implemented whenever there is uncertainty and doubt about the health and safety of students and staff.

If students and staff fear for their HEALTH and SAFETY, very little teaching and learning is going to occur in the building.

MODEL 4 (picture of students engaging in remote learning)

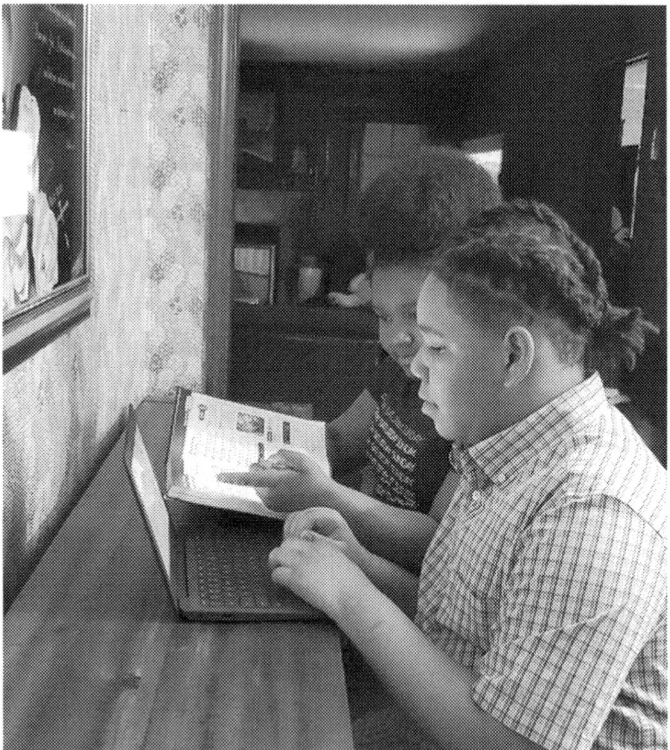

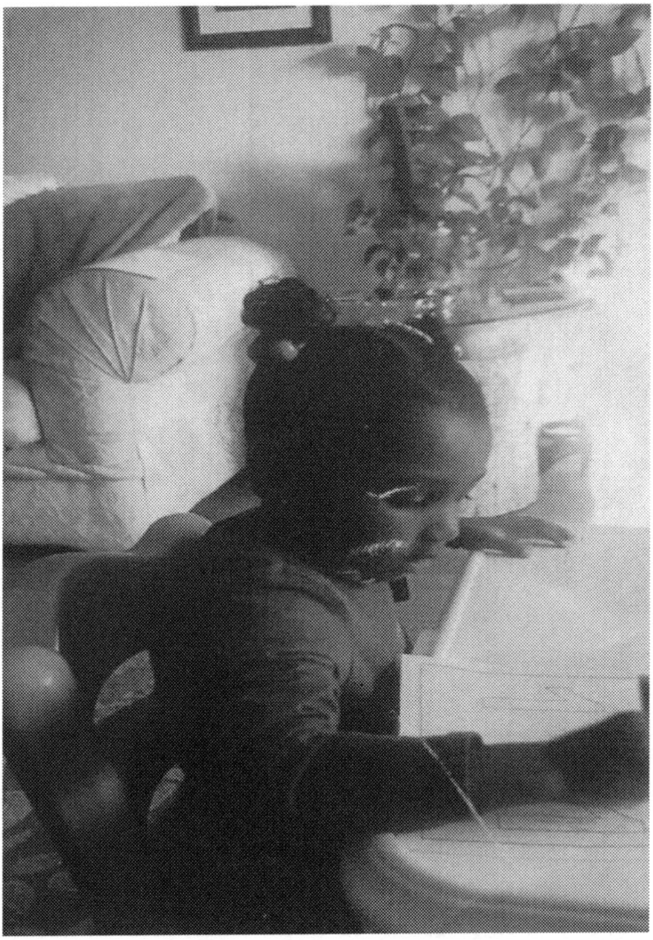

CHAPTER 7

HOW CAN WE MOVE BEYOND THE PANDEMIC?

This is an excellent question and totally understood. There is one word within the question that is critical to my response. That is the word CAN. To me, when you use the word CAN, it becomes a conversation about STRENGTH or POWER.

You can't move forward in HOURS, that would be too long. Try moving forward in minutes. Remember with the COVID-19, there was BREAKING NEWS every few minutes, so when we as a nation move forward, we must utilize minutes to move milestones. For example, you can say something like … "For the first 10-15 minutes, class, we are going to reflect upon our night and morning before we got to school …" Many schools already have similar activities. Then as you move through the day, present your lessons through an inquiry-based format.

Just as with the pandemic, everyone kept hoping that scientists would have the magic prescription of medication by the time we woke up, so give students similar challenges daily. You know why social media is so popular, it's mostly because of the challenges.

I remember giving my third graders at Sykuta Elementary School in Country Club Hills, Illinois, the challenge of creating a business that would benefit their community, by offering two or more services to working parents. Students had to construct prototypes of their creative businesses. The students did an outstanding job!!! They used math, science, and technology, and lots of reading to research and design these structures. I remember one business where parents could get their hair done, shop for groceries, all while leaving the children in a quality daycare center within the same facility. This was just one of the groups' creative models. Remember, this was a group of third graders!

Just allowing students to brainstorm and move outside of the four walls of traditional classrooms, motivated students to produce positive mindsets. Was it easy managing students within and outside of the four walls of my classroom? You know when I look back and reflect, it wasn't that difficult. I remember we set the rules and guidelines together and for the most part, they complied. The thrill on their faces as teachers and parents came to see presentations was so captivating. Parents would take pictures, along with me. This was so rewarding to the students. I still have the pictures of many of these projects saved on my Google drive!!!

So, what I am really saying is you start moving forward by the minutes, not by the hours, days, or weeks. You take care of the minutes and the hours, days, weeks, months, and years will follow. I'm reminded of my daily activities during the pandemic. At first, it was my location within the house after Illinois Governor J. B. Pritzker issued the 14-day stay-at-home order. Once that ended, again he added a 30-day stay-at-home order. The best way I mentally, physically and emotionally dealt with these orders was to simply take one day at a time, not 14 days, not 30 days, one day at a time. Even within that one day, I began to set a schedule of routines by the minutes. This made it so much easier to fathom what we, as a nation, were experiencing. Did it remove the problem at hand? No, it did not, but it boosted my mental energy to persevere and know that I am one of a resilient nation of people.

We would flatten the curve and get
to the other side together!!!

I think because I knew we were fighting this invisible enemy and at least 80% of the entire country were on the battlefield with me, I felt a remarkable inner strength from knowing that students, parents, teachers, administrators, boards of education, elected officials, first responders, doctors, nurses, scientists, engineers. ...you name it!!! Practically, everybody was pulling to end this pandemic!!! There is truly unity in community.

In the classroom, teachers must create visions that will spark challenges where students will want to contribute through thought-provoking conversations. Writing Prompt: Yes, we will survive the pandemic. Now what will we as students do to be more prepared if our country or one of our allies are attacked in a similar manner in the future? Since all students received equal access to this disaster, in some careful way, dialogue has to begin that will move us forward.

We must address the elephant in the room. Then we will begin the healing process. Until then, it remains an open sore. Individually, we must move towards inner peace. One person, one day at a time. You will get there.

CHAPTER 8

STEPS TO REACH NEW NORMALCY

Starting over is never an easy task. Thought must first prevail as to the destruction of what existed prior to the stage of wanting to push the reset button. However, in this case, we all recognize the need to begin again, but from a more determined state of mind, body, and soul. You see, having experienced a pandemic first hand touches the very core of our human existence. You live and breathe recycled thoughts. You begin to question your very existence and the struggle to survive mentally, physically, socially, emotionally, and spiritually. In the next breath, you begin to make connections to the hows and the whys that will push you forward to move on. But, remember, keep your eyes wide open.

More than anything, you begin to reach inside yourself for a sense of "back to normalcy". With no clear definition of what "normalcy" will look like, you begin by making giant baby steps. What this really means is you don't stand still. You reach out to family, friends, colleagues, neighbors, and all those who you were remotely connected to. They are still there, and they are reaching towards you. There is no shame in connecting with supporting individuals. The best way to begin is to breathe.

Step one is to reach out and find a productive friend to talk to. Students can find support through conversing with classmates, family, and friends who were already there before and during the pandemic. These relationships have already been established, but now since we have an additional piece added to our history, we should start building stronger and higher from this base.

Parents should accentuate relationships established through homeschooling and e-Learning. A boatload of parenting and educational support skills evolved almost overnight. Teachers, parents, and caregivers woke up to a new situation, and just had to make it work, and it did. I'm sure families were operating at a myriad of levels, but everyone kept it moving forward. Skill sets emerged from teachers as well as parents. Some parents probably felt overwhelmed by the Common Core State Standards and the underlying skills that students must master at their respective grade levels. Success rises from the ashes of many challenges, and surviving Pandemic 2020 is certainly a challenge for years to come.

The second step is to set immediate small goals you want to accomplish. This does not have to be anything long and drawn out. Having simple goals will make you want to jump out out bed and just get started. Of course you have long range goals in the back of your mind, but you don't want those goals to drive you. You will get there, but a mental overload can cause everything to come crashing down onto you. Remember, we are all resetting our lives. Set goals you can accomplish on your own and feel proud of. These little milestones that you reach each day will get you to the weeks, then months, and before you know it, a year will have elapsed since the onset of the pandemic.

The third step toward normalcy is to celebrate every success. Applaud yourself for the daily accomplishments. Administrators, recognize teachers and staff more often. Teachers, reward students for incremental accomplishments. It may seem like a very small reason to give a reward, but when moving away from the social and emotional pain of a pandemic, extrinsic rewards, prizes, and motivations will do so much for the young heart. I refer to this often as therapeutic teaching. Even the parents, guardians, teachers, school support staff will need the same kinds of rewards shown to them. Since we all had to go through it, let us all grow through it.

The final step towards normalcy is acknowledgement of process completion. You found a friend to share your success with. Next, you set a small reachable goal. Then, you celebrated completion of the goal. Finally, you validated your completion, usually by sharing with your friend, teacher, parent, colleague, the goal you accomplished, which will motivate you intrinsically to set a new goal for the next day.

Following these steps will incline all of us to achieve more while moving forward. We as a nation of students, parents, teachers, and citizens are resilient in nature; we will thrive, in spite of challenges. We will persevere because we can. We refuse to believe that any natural disaster, epidemic, or pandemic will destroy the energy that we have within. Through this inner strength, we will rise again, just as we did after other disasters, and we will be better and stronger together.

CHAPTER 9

ALL- INCLUSIVE VIRTUAL PARADIGM SHIFT

It has been the custom during my childhood, that at the start of a new school year, we all wait at the bus stop, get on the bus when it pulls up, look around and wave at our friends, unload when the bus arrives at the school, where we're directed to go to designated locations to meet our new homeroom teachers for the school year, and the academic school year progresses from there. But that was then, and up until the year 2019. However, the school year may look totally different in the Fall of 2020, for schools, academic centers, colleges, universities, and all institutions where populations of 15 or more students must congregate. Throughout the world, the pandemic has left a lasting impression, but not one that can't be masterminded successfully. We are a nation comprised of highly intellectual individuals.We don't wonder IF we can revitalize our educational structure for success, we say WHEN we re-ESTABLISH our educational system successfully.

There are four questions to guide your virtual paradigm shift. There is always a process that one must undergo in order to make a shift. Most of the time, extreme circumstances will cause things to shift. I'm sure everyone will agree that a pandemic registers as an extreme occurrence. Therefore, after a disaster of this magnitude, there will be a number of shifts, but we must pivot our energies in a direction of progress and forward motions. You tell yourself daily, "Today I am here, but tomorrow I will be there". You are setting and reaching small milestones daily.

Start with these four questions:

The first question is "DID I INCLUDE OR MAKE PROVISIONS FOR EVERYONE?" One thing the entire world should have come to grips with is the fact that **We Are All Important**... every baby, child, adult, parent, neighbor, co-worker, employee, employer, supervisor, front line worker, first responder, and patient in the hospital. We don't want to make a habit of allowing students, friends, family, neighbors, and others, feel less than or simply put, left out. This is so critical for our very young, the disabled, minorities, and our disadvantaged populations. No person wants to feel isolated. Inside of community, we see the word unity. Don't ever overlook that vital part.

The second question is "CAN EVERYBODY SEE ME?" You see, in this new normalcy, it might sound crazy, but unless you're about to commit a crime, you want to be seen. There is safety within vision. Teachers want students to see their demonstrations of how to solve problems or write a convincing persuasive essay, whether through traditional or virtual learning. Students want teachers to see their work, for providing corrective feedback. Employees want employers to see when workplace is not safe or they feel threatened, small children in daycare centers where parents can view their children from their workplace and rest assured seeing virtually, they are safe, riders on public transit want security officers to intercede when the patrons' safety is being jeopardized, in politics, and I could go on and on, but my point remains. CAN EVERYBODY SEE ME? This is the second step towards an all-inclusive virtual paradigm shift.

The third question, equally important, is "AM I ON TASK?" I can imagine that you are thinking, "I don't want my teacher, my mom or dad, my boss, or my superior knowing whether I'm on task or not, but in reality, you actually do. Let me explain. If you are at school virtually and your teacher is tallying grades, emails you and ask you to submit your work electronically, but all morning you were playing a video game, or sleeping excessively late, you missed the ZOOM lesson the teacher provided, where she explicitly demonstrated the strategy, other students who were on task practiced, asked questions, received clarity, while you were off-task. So, now it's time to submit your work. This is just one example in the school framework of why it's good to stay on task. It is absolutely just as vital in the workplace. One employee off-task could cost a company thousands of dollars in loss revenue and productivity. For example, if your company is manufacturing car parts, but when it's time to submit a massive order, the parts aren't ready, because you have wasted an enormous amount of time on your cellphone during times when you were suppose to be mass producing the product, the buyer will look for another supplier whose employees are able to deliver the services or products. These are just two examples of the importance of on-task behavior.

The final question is "AM I GROWING THROUGH WHAT I'M GOING THROUGH?.

Now this question is key for advancement in your life. Can I show you that I'm growing? Even though you're in California and I'm in Illinois, can you take a look at my growth? How is my work looking? I must begin to embrace every victory, whether large or small. Virtually, I want to be able to connect with peers, colleagues, employees, employers, business interests across the globe, because another lesson from the pandemic is that progress knows no boundaries. We must learn to search for answers and solutions seamlessly. This new virtual platform is a reality that we all must embrace. Even if we begin with baby steps, just keep moving forward. Technology is here to stay. Let it productively become one of your BFF's!

CHAPTER 10

ALIGNING THE HOME FOR VIRTUAL ACADEMIC EXCELLENCE

How do you set up your home environment for virtual academic excellence? You want your home to radiate as a learning institution supplanting what was once deemed as "homework ". Since schools are being redeveloped to meet the needs of the new America, beyond Pandemic 2020, the home culture has to mirror the educational shift.

For all the parents and families who have been

homeschooling prior to the pandemic, the picture won't necessarily relate as specific to you, however, for the rest of America, this is a huge undertaking- REMOTE LEARNING. The first step towards moving forward is acknowledging where we are, The good news is you are in the midst of surviving a pandemic. With the right mindset, you will evolve stronger and better as parents and guardians.

At this point, we must pull ourselves up by our bootstraps with our hands on technology, and our eyes on platforms that will transform our destiny. For quite sometime, we've heard the expression that there's a lot of information "out there". We can no longer allow pertinent and relevant information to be "out there". We must use every day and every muscle within ourselves to gather and internalize the information that's "out there" in meaningful ways.

How do we accomplish this? Parents and guardians must set daily learning goals. Once these goals are met, we must celebrate along the way but keep moving forward.

For example, since I live in the state of Illinois, today I want my son to begin researching the state's capital. Tomorrow, we'll probably move to largest cities or other aspects of the state, like natural resources, but by this weekend, my son will have very strong background knowledge about the state of Illinois. Could this assignment extend into two weeks? Most definitely. Through Google, you could extend it based on the comprehension and the level of complexity the assignment presents for your child. Parents and guardians can CONTROL ACADEMIC VICTORIES FOR THEIR CHILDREN. Living in the city of Chicago affords parents with a rich history of research ideas and topics.There are individuals associated with the state of Illinois and the city of Chicago, opening the doors for tons of research to be done. A mind is still a terrible thing to waste! When I think about the Great Chicago Fire, the Sears Tower, Navy Pier, Dr. Daniel Hale Williams, Barack and Michelle Obama, Harold Washington, Michael Jordan, Dr. Bernard Fantus, Gwendolyn Brooks, Harrison Ford, Ida B. Wells, Emmett Till, Wrigley Field, just to name a few of the possible research topics … there is so much history!!! This, my friends, is VIRTUAL LEARNING.

Research using all the tools you have available, formulating questions along the way, revisiting history, making history, pursuing learning at levels far superior to students who woke up late, found a snack, and grabbed a video game controller. We must prepare for this new America! The students who capitalize and make use of valuable learning opportunities will be rewarded accordingly. Virtual learning is advanced in comparison to traditional acquisition of knowledge, and yet it's just a click away.

You see, here's the reality. No one should come to your country today, start studying your history, and next week, know more about your history than you do. It just should not happen. If you're going to compete in a global society, you can't just have ownership of a chrome book, laptop, iPhone, and reign supreme. There are libraries of information stored inside of these devices. However, you must have an acquisition plan for becoming successful. You won't just wake up one morning smarter and stronger. Perseverance and determination are key competencies that you must possess.

Regardless of what you're feeling right now, this can be A BEAUTIFUL WORLD. Get to know it, one continent at a time, or a mixture, just keep it moving. We learned quite a bit about the Spanish Flu of 1918 because of the Pandemic of 2020. Something is wrong with that picture! What I am saying is, that is an example of reactive learning. We need to steer our young minds towards proactive learning or productive research. How many years have elapsed between 1918 and 2020? There is SOOOO MUCH history between those years. Right now, we are still in this war with an invisible enemy. Here's another example. Let's look at a few other wars the United States have been involved in. How much did the Vietnam War cost the United States of America?

What was the dollar amount? How many lives were lost? Never stop learning. Life is a cycle of continuous learning!

This will enable you to achieve and control victory beyond COVID-19. You are possibly wondering for a few reasons. First, you must be thinking where can we find a victory in the midst of a pandemic. Secondly, the question probably is how can you control a victory, Then, it brings you to the idea of moving "beyond" the pandemic. You see, when I think about the entire United States of America prior to the pandemic, in my mind, it's like a different age. I have begun to refer to that America as America 1.0. But since the pandemic has occurred, to me, this is now America 2.0. These two ages in history can't exist concurrently, meaning, if America 2.0 is present, then America 1.0 no longer exists.

So, when you allow your mind to conceptualize the two Americas, it will bring you to a place of preparation, peace, and power. This journey hasn't been an easy one, but it is a trek we must embark upon. First, let me elaborate on the three P's: Preparation, Peace, and Power. We must prepare our lives differently. What worked during America 1.0, in our daily lives, may not sustain us in America 2.0. At times, some things may work out, but on a larger scale, many things may have to be improvised. For example, the institution of schooling, where the parents sent the kids to school and the breadwinner or parent was off to work, this picture may have a whole new, innovative look during America 2.0. Some adult or caregiver may need to be home all day because younger children will require their presence for remote learning, parenting, nutritional, social, and emotional support. Services that once occurred at a tradition school building may now be requirements for the home environment. One takeaway from the pandemic is that students can still thrive and teachers can still teach with the anchor of a technology- driven support system. The overarching level of preparation has to be guided by a success mindset.

You know I was on the inside looking out, working as a mentor for new teachers when COVID-19 became apparent. Let me first acknowledge the superb job of the teachers I mentored in Hazel Crest, Illinois. Without hesitation, they never missed a beat in stepping up to provide instruction to students, continuing with the Common Core State Standards, providing instructional virtual supports through ZOOM lessons, KAMI, GOOGLE Classroom,

Google Docs, Google Slides, Discovery Education, Legends of Learning, TIME For Kids, See Saw, Lalilo, Freckles, KAHOOT, Teachers provided a deluge of remote learning supports so that students wouldn't just keep up, but they would feel challenged to excel, through research assignments and other student-produced performance products, such as videos, power points, slide presentations, research reports, and so forth. This is just one example of the preparedness we move forward with. In the employer/employee relationships across the country, employers realized that many employees who are making the 1-2 hour transports to work could possibly be more productive just logging in from home.

I was working as a mentor to new teachers when COVID-19 happened. I could have panicked and just lost it, but I realized that this was the beginning of a shift from the old into the new. I was accustomed to going into the classrooms of first year teachers supporting them. This was, in summary, my job description. But now, after the governor of Illinois, and governors across the country, began to shut down schools and stay-at-home orders were issued, whereas I was mentoring teachers, what would I do now? How would I provide support to teachers from my home? Even more, how would teachers reach all of their students, since some didn't have the technology tools they needed to jump into remote learning without notice. I began to look at my home computer through new lens. I quickly realized that it embodied the elements I needed to fulfill my obligation of supporting the new teachers of this school district. However, my heart was deeply saddened because I realized not every student would have the electronic edge they would need to keep up and some parents would have to make tough decisions about their jobs, careers, and families. I did every thing I could to provide support to the new teachers, learning and growing together. We had to make it work, for the children! To make sure students were learning, remember, you can always ask them and rely on their answers. I jumped on the ZOOM platform and continued providing support to teachers. The relationships teachers built with students early on was so critical in sustaining everyone as the school year successfully ended in May. This experience caused me to revisit the poem that I wrote in 2009:

(POEM)

"YES, YOU CAN!!!"

Don't underestimate your power,

You are as strong as the wind;

Don't be fooled by put-downs,

Your wings aren't that thin!

Fly as high as an eagle,

Yes, I said, You Can.

Just mount up and soar

Like the lion, you have a mighty roar!

Take life by the horns,

There is purpose for which we all were born

Believe me when I say …

For those challenges

Facing you today …

Stand Tall and Know,

Each Day as You Grow,

YES, YOU CAN!!!

BIBLIOGRAPHY

Fullan, M. G. (1991). *The new meaning of educational change.* New York: Teachers College Press.

Jacobson, J., Olsen, C., Rice, J.K., Sweetland, S., & Ralph, J. (2001).*Educational achievement and black-white inequality.* Washington, DC: National Center for Educational Statistics.

Lezotte, L. (1997). *Learning for all: What will it take?* Okemos, MI: Effective Schools Products, Ltd.

Wiley, V. (2020). *Quality teaching -Beating the odds for at-risk students.* Bloomington, IN:Westbow Press

THOUGHTS TO PONDER

One major concern for me is the fact that we never want to deliberately return to a phase in education where we're so driven by state -mandated assessments, that we ignore the human element. After speaking to students across the country, the echo was "Thank God, we don't have to take those state tests!" It became so apparent to me, the overwhelming level of anxiety our students faced, because of traditional schooling. Somewhere lost in all of this is the fact that school should be a place where students thrive and are excited about learning in a safe environment.

Parents and guardians, you must always be

the most vocal advocate for your child. Here's a thought- How much screen time is safe for your child? Research, parents, and make sure there is a balance in your child's life. Be smart. Stay informed. Be relentless living in the "know". Continue building strong relationships. Teachers must remain the heroes for all students. Lawmakers, become the anchor that parents, teachers, and communities can rely on due to your never-ending quest to provide funding so that we will be one nation, providing liberty and justice for all, funding education equitably. It is my sincere desire that we can initiate that through America 2.0-VIRTUAL LEARNING- Reaching and Teaching ALL OF OUR STUDENTS BY ANY MEANS NECESSARY, far BEYOND PANDEMIC 2020!!!

NEXT LEVEL TEACHING!!!

Printed in the United States
By Bookmasters